Mindfulness and Progressive Supranuclear Palsy: Techniques for Coping

Laura Louizos

DEDICATION

To all those affected by Progressive Supranuclear Palsy (PSP) – the patients who face each day with courage, the caregivers who provide unwavering support, and the families who share the journey.

This book is especially dedicated to my mother, whose strength and grace inspired every page. Your spirit lives on in the lives you touched and the love you shared.

And to all the caregivers who tirelessly give of themselves, your compassion and resilience are the true essence of mindfulness in action. May this book provide you with the tools, support, and inspiration you need to continue your journey with hope and peace.

TABLE OF CONTENTS

Disclaimer: Medical Advice

The information provided in this book, "Mindfulness and Progressive Supranuclear Palsy: Techniques for Coping," is intended for educational and informational purposes only. It is not a substitute for professional medical advice, diagnosis, or treatment. Always seek the advice of your physician or other qualified health providers with any questions you may have regarding a medical condition.

- **Consult with Professionals:** The mindfulness practices and techniques described in this book are not intended to replace the advice and care of medical professionals. If you or a loved one has been diagnosed with Progressive Supranuclear Palsy (PSP) or any other medical condition, consult with your healthcare provider before starting any new treatment or exercise program.

- **Individual Differences:** The experiences and outcomes described in the personal stories and testimonials in this book are specific to those individuals. Results may vary, and what works for one person may not work for another. Always tailor mindfulness practices to suit your personal needs and circumstances.

- **Emergency Situations:** Do not disregard or delay seeking professional medical advice because of information read in this book. In case of a medical

emergency, call your doctor or emergency
services immediately.

- **No Endorsement:** The mention of specific
  products, websites, or services in this book does
  not imply endorsement. The resources and
  references provided are for informational
  purposes only and are based on available
  information at the time of writing.

- **Updates and Changes:** Medical knowledge and
  practices are continually evolving. While we strive
  to provide accurate and up-to-date information,
  the content of this book may become outdated or
  inaccurate over time. Always refer to current
  medical guidelines and consult with healthcare
  professionals for the most recent and relevant
  information.

By using this book, you acknowledge and agree to this
disclaimer and understand that the authors and
publishers are not responsible for any outcomes
resulting from the use of the information provided.

Chapter 1: Introduction to Mindfulness

1.1 What is Mindfulness?

Mindfulness is the practice of being fully present and engaged in the current moment, without judgment. It involves paying close attention to your thoughts, feelings, bodily sensations, and the surrounding environment. This practice has roots in ancient meditation traditions but has been widely adopted in modern psychology and wellness practices for its numerous benefits.

For individuals living with Progressive Supranuclear Palsy (PSP) and their caregivers, mindfulness can offer a way to manage stress, reduce anxiety, and improve overall well-being. By focusing on the present moment, you can better handle the challenges and unpredictability of daily life with PSP.

1.2 The Benefits of Mindfulness for PSP Patients and Caregivers

Mindfulness offers a range of benefits that can be particularly valuable for PSP patients and their caregivers:

- **Reduced Stress and Anxiety:** Mindfulness helps to calm the mind and reduce the physical and emotional symptoms of stress and anxiety. This can lead to a more peaceful and manageable daily experience.

- **Improved Emotional Regulation:** By observing thoughts and feelings without immediate reaction, individuals can develop better emotional regulation, leading to fewer emotional outbursts and a more stable mood.
- **Enhanced Focus and Clarity:** Practicing mindfulness can improve concentration and mental clarity, making it easier to handle tasks and decisions that arise throughout the day.
- **Better Coping Skills:** Mindfulness encourages acceptance and non-judgmental awareness, helping individuals cope with difficult emotions and challenging situations more effectively.
- **Increased Physical Relaxation:** Techniques such as mindful breathing and body scans can help reduce physical tension and pain, promoting relaxation and better sleep.

1.3 Setting Realistic Expectations

While mindfulness offers numerous benefits, it's important to set realistic expectations, especially when dealing with a complex condition like PSP. Here are some key points to consider:

- **Start Small:** Begin with short, simple mindfulness practices. Even a few minutes a day can make a difference.
- **Be Patient:** Progress may be slow and incremental. Be patient with yourself and your

loved ones as you integrate mindfulness into your daily routine.

- **Customize Your Practice:** Adapt mindfulness techniques to suit your specific needs and capabilities. What works for one person may not work for another.
- **Focus on the Present:** Avoid using mindfulness as a way to escape from the challenges of PSP. Instead, use it as a tool to better engage with and manage those challenges.
- **Seek Support:** Consider joining mindfulness groups or seeking guidance from a mindfulness teacher, especially if you or your loved one is new to the practice.

By embracing mindfulness, PSP patients and caregivers can cultivate a greater sense of calm, resilience, and well-being. The following chapters will provide practical techniques and exercises to help you get started on this journey.

Chapter 2: Getting Started with Mindfulness

2.1 Creating a Mindful Environment

Creating a conducive environment for mindfulness practice is crucial. A peaceful and comfortable space can enhance your mindfulness experience, helping you to relax and focus.

- **Choose a Quiet Space:** Find a quiet place in your home where you can practice without interruptions. This could be a corner of a room, a comfortable chair, or even a spot in your garden.
- **Comfort is Key:** Ensure you have comfortable seating, whether it's a cushion on the floor, a chair, or a recliner. Use blankets or pillows to support your body and make the space cozy.
- **Minimize Distractions:** Turn off electronic devices or put them on silent. If possible, dim the lights or use natural lighting to create a soothing atmosphere.
- **Personal Touch:** Add personal items that promote relaxation, such as candles, incense, soft music, or nature sounds. Some people find it helpful to have a focal point, like a plant or a calming picture.

2.2 Basic Mindfulness Techniques

Starting with basic mindfulness techniques can help you build a solid foundation for your practice. Here are a few simple exercises to get you started:

- **Mindful Breathing:** Sit comfortably and close your eyes. Focus on your breath as you inhale and exhale naturally. Notice the sensation of the breath entering and leaving your body. If your mind wanders, gently bring your focus back to your breath.
- **Body Scan:** Lie down or sit comfortably. Starting from your toes and moving up to your head, bring your attention to each part of your body. Notice any sensations, tension, or relaxation. Don't try to change anything; simply observe.
- **Mindful Observation:** Choose an object in your environment, such as a flower or a piece of artwork. Spend a few minutes observing it closely, noticing its colors, shapes, textures, and any other details. This exercise helps to anchor your mind in the present moment.

2.3 Establishing a Daily Practice

Consistency is key to reaping the benefits of mindfulness. Establishing a daily practice can help make mindfulness a natural part of your routine.

- **Set Aside Time:** Dedicate a specific time each day for mindfulness practice. It could be in the morning to start your day calmly, during a break, or before bedtime to unwind.
- **Start Small:** Begin with short sessions, such as 5 to 10 minutes. Gradually increase the duration as you become more comfortable with the practice.

- **Be Flexible:** While consistency is important, it's also essential to be flexible. If you miss a session, don't be hard on yourself. Simply start again the next day.
- **Use Reminders:** Set reminders on your phone or write notes to remind yourself to practice mindfulness. Over time, it will become a natural part of your daily routine.
- **Journal Your Experience:** Keep a mindfulness journal to record your experiences, thoughts, and any changes you notice in your mood and well-being. This can help you track your progress and stay motivated.

By creating a mindful environment, practicing basic techniques, and establishing a daily routine, you'll lay the groundwork for a successful mindfulness practice. The next chapter will delve deeper into specific breathing exercises that can further enhance your mindfulness journey.

Chapter 3: Breathing Exercises

3.1 The Power of Breath

Breathing is a fundamental aspect of mindfulness. It serves as an anchor to keep you grounded in the present moment. Conscious breathing can help regulate the nervous system, reduce stress, and promote relaxation. For PSP patients and caregivers, mastering breathing exercises can provide a powerful tool for managing anxiety and enhancing overall well-being.

3.2 Simple Breathing Techniques

1. **Deep Belly Breathing:**

   - **Step 1:** Sit or lie down in a comfortable position. Place one hand on your chest and the other on your belly.
   - **Step 2:** Take a slow, deep breath in through your nose, allowing your belly to rise as it fills with air. Your chest should remain relatively still.
   - **Step 3:** Exhale slowly through your mouth, feeling your belly fall. Repeat this process for a few minutes, focusing on the rise and fall of your belly.

2. **4-7-8 Breathing:**
   - **Step 1:** Sit comfortably with your back straight.

- **Step 2:** Inhale quietly through your nose for a count of 4.
- **Step 3:** Hold your breath for a count of 7.
- **Step 4:** Exhale completely through your mouth for a count of 8. Repeat this cycle four times, gradually increasing the number of cycles as you become more comfortable.

3. **Box Breathing (Square Breathing):**

- **Step 1:** Sit in a comfortable position.
- **Step 2:** Inhale through your nose for a count of 4.
- **Step 3:** Hold your breath for a count of 4.
- **Step 4:** Exhale through your mouth for a count of 4.
- **Step 5:** Hold your breath again for a count of 4. Repeat this process for several cycles, focusing on maintaining a steady rhythm.

3.3 Guided Breathing Practices

Guided breathing practices can provide structure and support, making it easier to maintain focus and relaxation.

1. **Guided Audio Sessions:**

- There are many guided breathing sessions available online through apps or websites. These sessions typically involve a soothing voice guiding you through various breathing techniques, often accompanied by calming music or nature sounds.

2. **Visualization Breathing:**
   - **Step 1:** Sit comfortably and close your eyes.
   - **Step 2:** As you inhale, visualize a wave of calm energy entering your body, filling you with peace and relaxation.
   - **Step 3:** As you exhale, imagine any tension or stress leaving your body, carried away by the breath.
   - **Step 4:** Continue this visualization for several minutes, focusing on the calming imagery and sensations.

3. **Breathing Apps:**
   - Numerous apps are designed to assist with breathing exercises, offering visual guides, timers, and customizable sessions. Examples include Calm, Headspace, and Breathe2Relax. These tools can be particularly helpful for PSP patients and caregivers who prefer structured guidance.

By practicing these breathing exercises regularly, PSP patients and caregivers can harness the power of breath to manage stress, improve emotional regulation, and enhance overall well-being. The next chapter will explore meditation practices that complement these breathing techniques, offering additional tools for mindfulness and relaxation.

Chapter 4: Meditation Practices

4.1 Introduction to Meditation

Meditation is a practice that involves focusing the mind and eliminating distractions to achieve a state of mental clarity and emotional calm. For PSP patients and caregivers, meditation can be a valuable tool to manage stress, improve concentration, and foster a sense of peace. By incorporating meditation into your routine, you can enhance your overall well-being and better cope with the challenges of PSP.

4.2 Types of Meditation

1. **Mindfulness Meditation:**
   - **Purpose:** Cultivates awareness of the present moment.
   - **Practice:** Sit comfortably, close your eyes, and focus on your breath. Notice your thoughts and sensations without judgment. If your mind wanders, gently bring your focus back to your breath.
2. **Loving-Kindness Meditation (Metta):**
   - **Purpose:** Fosters compassion and love towards oneself and others.
   - **Practice:** Sit comfortably and close your eyes. Repeat phrases such as "May I be happy, may I be healthy, may I be safe, may I live with ease." Gradually extend these

wishes to others, including loved ones and even those you find challenging.

3. **Body Scan Meditation:**
   - **Purpose:** Enhances body awareness and relaxation.
   - **Practice:** Lie down or sit comfortably. Close your eyes and bring your attention to different parts of your body, starting from your toes and moving up to your head. Notice any sensations, tension, or relaxation.

4. **Guided Visualization:**
   - **Purpose:** Uses imagery to promote relaxation and mental clarity.
   - **Practice:** Sit or lie down comfortably and close your eyes. Listen to a guided meditation that takes you through a peaceful scene, such as a beach or forest. Visualize the details vividly, engaging all your senses.

5. **Chanting or Mantra Meditation:**
   - **Purpose:** Focuses the mind through repetitive sound or phrases.
   - **Practice:** Sit comfortably and choose a word or phrase (mantra) to repeat, such as "Om" or "Peace." Repeat the mantra silently or aloud, focusing on its sound and vibration.

4.3 Guided Meditation for Relaxation

Guided meditation can be particularly helpful for beginners or those who prefer structure. Here are some steps to follow for a guided relaxation meditation:

1. **Find a Comfortable Position:**
   - Sit or lie down in a comfortable position. Ensure your body is supported and relaxed.
2. **Close Your Eyes:**
   - Close your eyes to minimize distractions and focus inward.
3. **Focus on Your Breath:**
   - Take a few deep breaths, inhaling through your nose and exhaling through your mouth. Allow your breath to settle into a natural rhythm.
4. **Listen to the Guide:**
   - Choose a guided meditation recording or app. Listen to the guide's voice as they lead you through a relaxation process. Follow their instructions, focusing on your breath, body sensations, or visualizations.
5. **Let Go of Tension:**
   - As you follow the guided meditation, consciously release any tension or stress in your body. Visualize your muscles relaxing and your mind becoming calm.

6. **Stay Present:**
   - If your mind wanders, gently bring your focus back to the guide's voice and the sensations in your body.
7. **Gradually Return:**
   - When the guided meditation ends, take a few moments to slowly bring your awareness back to the present. Open your eyes and take note of how you feel.

Regular practice of these meditation techniques can significantly enhance your ability to cope with the emotional and physical challenges of PSP. The next chapter will focus on body awareness and movement practices, providing additional tools to support your mindfulness journey.

Chapter 5: Body Awareness and Movement

5.1 Mindful Movement

Mindful movement integrates physical activity with mindfulness practices, promoting body awareness, relaxation, and overall well-being. For PSP patients and caregivers, gentle and intentional movements can improve flexibility, reduce tension, and enhance the mind-body connection.

5.2 Gentle Yoga and Stretching

Yoga and stretching exercises can be adapted to suit various physical abilities, making them accessible for both PSP patients and caregivers. These practices help to increase flexibility, improve circulation, and promote relaxation.

1. **Seated Yoga Poses:**
   - **Cat-Cow Stretch:**
     - Sit on a chair with your feet flat on the floor. Place your hands on your knees.
     - Inhale, arch your back, and look up (Cow Pose).
     - Exhale, round your back, and tuck your chin towards your chest (Cat Pose).
     - Repeat for several breaths.

- **Seated Forward Bend:**
  - Sit on a chair with your feet flat on the floor.
  - Inhale, lengthen your spine.
  - Exhale, hinge at your hips, and lean forward, reaching towards your toes. Only go as far as comfortable.
  - Hold for a few breaths, then slowly rise back up.
- **Neck Stretches:**
  - Sit comfortably and keep your back straight.
  - Gently tilt your head to the right, bringing your right ear towards your right shoulder.
  - Hold for a few breaths, then switch sides.

2. **Standing Yoga Poses (with Support):**
   - **Mountain Pose:**
     - Stand with your feet hip-width apart, arms at your sides.
     - Press your feet firmly into the ground, engage your legs, and lengthen your spine.
     - Relax your shoulders and take deep breaths.
   - **Supported Tree Pose:**
     - Stand with your feet hip-width apart.
     - Hold onto a chair or wall for support.

- Shift your weight onto your left foot
  and place the sole of your right foot
  on your inner left thigh or calf (avoid
  the knee).
- Bring your hands to your heart or
  hold onto the support.
- Hold for a few breaths, then switch
  sides.

3. **Gentle Stretching:**
   - **Hamstring Stretch:**
     - Sit on the edge of a chair with one leg
       extended straight in front of you,
       heel on the floor.
     - Keep your back straight and hinge at
       your hips to lean forward slightly.
     - Hold for a few breaths, then switch
       legs.
   - **Shoulder Stretch:**
     - Sit or stand comfortably.
     - Bring your right arm across your
       chest and hold it with your left hand.
     - Hold for a few breaths, then switch
       arms.

5.3 Body Scan Meditation

Body scan meditation is a technique that promotes
relaxation and body awareness by focusing attention on
different parts of the body. This practice can help reduce
tension, manage pain, and enhance the connection
between mind and body.

1. **Preparation:**
   - Find a comfortable position, either lying down or sitting in a chair. Close your eyes and take a few deep breaths to settle into the practice.
2. **Begin the Scan:**
   - Start with your toes. Focus your attention on the sensations in your toes. Notice any tension, tingling, warmth, or relaxation.
   - Gradually move your attention up through your feet, ankles, and legs. Spend a few moments on each area, observing without judgment.
3. **Continue Upward:**
   - Move your focus through your hips, lower back, and abdomen. Notice any areas of discomfort or relaxation.
   - Continue to your chest, upper back, and shoulders. Observe the sensations and let go of any tension with each exhale.
4. **Upper Body:**
   - Focus on your arms, hands, and fingers. Notice the sensations in each part.
   - Move your attention to your neck, throat, and jaw. Relax these areas as you breathe.
5. **Head and Face:**
   - Finally, focus on your face, including your eyes, forehead, and scalp. Notice any tension or relaxation.
   - Spend a few moments observing the overall sensations in your body.

6. **Finish:**

- When you are ready, slowly bring your attention back to the room. Open your eyes and take a moment to notice how you feel.

Incorporating mindful movement and body awareness practices into your daily routine can significantly enhance your physical and mental well-being. The next chapter will explore techniques for coping with stress and anxiety, providing further tools to support you on your journey.

Chapter 6: Coping with Stress and Anxiety

6.1 Understanding Stress and Anxiety in PSP

Living with Progressive Supranuclear Palsy (PSP) can bring about significant stress and anxiety for both patients and caregivers. Understanding these emotions is the first step toward managing them effectively.

- **Stress:** A natural response to challenging situations, stress can manifest physically, emotionally, and mentally. For PSP patients, stress may arise from managing symptoms, treatment regimens, and the uncertainty of the disease progression. Caregivers may experience stress from the demands of providing constant care and the emotional toll of witnessing a loved one's decline.
- **Anxiety:** Often linked with stress, anxiety involves persistent worry and fear about future events. PSP patients might feel anxious about their health and independence, while caregivers may worry about their ability to provide adequate care and the future of their loved one.

Recognizing the signs of stress and anxiety—such as irritability, fatigue, difficulty concentrating, and physical symptoms like headaches or muscle tension—is crucial in addressing these issues.

6.2 Mindfulness Techniques for Stress Reduction

1. **Grounding Exercises:**
   - **Five Senses Exercise:**
     - Sit comfortably and take a few deep breaths.
     - Focus on each of your five senses one by one: What are five things you can see? Four things you can touch? Three things you can hear? Two things you can smell? One thing you can taste?
     - This exercise helps anchor you in the present moment and reduces anxiety.
2. **Progressive Muscle Relaxation:**
   - **Step 1:** Find a comfortable position and close your eyes.
   - **Step 2:** Starting with your toes, tense the muscles in your feet for a few seconds, then release.
   - **Step 3:** Gradually move up your body, tensing and relaxing each muscle group (legs, abdomen, chest, arms, and face).
   - **Step 4:** Focus on the sensation of relaxation after releasing each muscle group.
3. **Visualization Techniques:**
   - **Calm Place Visualization:**
     - Sit or lie down comfortably and close your eyes.

- Imagine a place where you feel completely calm and safe. It could be a real place or a fantasy location.
- Engage all your senses to make the visualization vivid: notice the sights, sounds, smells, and sensations.
- Spend a few minutes in this calming place, allowing yourself to relax and unwind.

6.3 Practical Tips for Managing Anxiety

1. **Routine and Structure:**
   - **Create a Daily Schedule:** Establishing a routine can provide a sense of stability and predictability, reducing anxiety.
   - **Break Tasks into Manageable Steps:** Large tasks can be overwhelming. Breaking them down into smaller, more manageable steps can make them less daunting.
2. **Healthy Lifestyle Choices:**
   - **Exercise Regularly:** Physical activity can reduce stress hormones and trigger the release of endorphins, improving mood and energy levels.
   - **Eat a Balanced Diet:** Proper nutrition supports overall health and can influence mood and energy levels.
   - **Prioritize Sleep:** Quality sleep is essential for managing stress and anxiety. Establish a

regular sleep routine and create a restful sleep environment.

3. **Social Support:**
   - **Connect with Others:** Talking to friends, family, or support groups can provide emotional support and practical advice.
   - **Seek Professional Help:** If anxiety becomes overwhelming, consider talking to a mental health professional who can offer strategies and support.

4. **Mindfulness and Relaxation Practices:**
   - **Practice Regularly:** Incorporate mindfulness and relaxation techniques into your daily routine to build resilience against stress and anxiety.
   - **Be Patient:** Developing new habits takes time. Be patient with yourself as you integrate these practices into your life.

By incorporating these techniques and practical tips, PSP patients and caregivers can better manage stress and anxiety, improving their overall quality of life. The next chapter will explore mindful communication, offering tools to enhance understanding and connection in relationships.

Chapter 7: Mindful Communication

7.1 The Importance of Communication

Effective communication is vital for PSP patients and their caregivers. It ensures that needs are met, emotions are expressed, and support is provided. Mindful communication involves being fully present during interactions, listening actively, and responding with empathy and clarity. This approach can significantly improve relationships and reduce misunderstandings and frustrations.

7.2 Mindful Listening

1. **Be Present:**
   - **Focus on the Speaker:** Give your full attention to the person speaking. Put away distractions such as phones or other devices.
   - **Maintain Eye Contact:** This shows that you are engaged and interested in what the other person is saying.
2. **Active Listening Techniques:**
   - **Reflective Listening:** Paraphrase what the speaker has said to show that you understand. For example, "It sounds like you're feeling frustrated because..."

- **Ask Open-Ended Questions:** Encourage the speaker to share more by asking questions that require more than a yes or no answer. For example, "How did that make you feel?" or "Can you tell me more about that?"

3. **Empathy and Validation:**
   - **Show Empathy:** Try to understand the speaker's perspective and emotions. You can say things like, "I can see how that would be difficult for you."
   - **Validate Feelings:** Acknowledge the speaker's feelings without judgment. For example, "It's okay to feel upset about this."

7.3 Expressing Needs and Emotions

1. **Use "I" Statements:**
   - **Express Your Feelings:** Use "I" statements to express your feelings without blaming or criticizing. For example, "I feel overwhelmed when I don't get help with the daily tasks."
   - **Be Specific:** Clearly state your needs and what you would like to happen. For example, "I need help with preparing meals because it's becoming difficult for me to manage alone."

2. **Be Honest and Direct:**
   - **Communicate Clearly:** Speak openly about your feelings and needs. Avoid vague or indirect statements that can lead to misunderstandings.
   - **Stay Calm and Respectful:** Even when discussing difficult topics, aim to remain calm and respectful. This helps to keep the conversation productive.
3. **Set Boundaries:**
   - **Know Your Limits:** Recognize your own limits and communicate them clearly. For example, "I need some time to rest after lunch because I feel exhausted."
   - **Respect Others' Boundaries:** Be mindful of the other person's boundaries as well. Respect their need for space or time to process information.

7.4 Resolving Conflicts Mindfully

1. **Stay Calm:**
   - **Take a Break if Needed:** If a conversation becomes heated, take a moment to breathe and calm down before continuing.
   - **Use Relaxation Techniques:** Practice deep breathing or other relaxation techniques to stay calm during conflicts.
2. **Listen and Reflect:**
   - **Listen to Understand:** Focus on understanding the other person's

perspective rather than preparing your response.

- **Reflect and Validate:** Reflect back what you've heard and validate their feelings. This shows that you respect their viewpoint even if you don't agree.

3. **Find Common Ground:**
   - **Identify Shared Goals:** Look for common goals or interests that can serve as a foundation for finding a solution.
   - **Collaborate on Solutions:** Work together to find a solution that satisfies both parties. Be willing to compromise and explore different options.

4. **Forgive and Move On:**
   - **Let Go of Grudges:** Holding onto resentment can damage relationships. Practice forgiveness and let go of past grievances.
   - **Focus on the Present:** Concentrate on moving forward and building a positive relationship.

By practicing mindful communication, PSP patients and caregivers can enhance their relationships, ensure that their needs are met, and create a supportive environment. The next chapter will explore techniques to enhance emotional well-being, providing further tools to support your mindfulness journey.

Chapter 8: Enhancing Emotional Well-Being

8.1 Recognizing and Accepting Emotions

Emotional well-being is crucial for both PSP patients and caregivers. Recognizing and accepting your emotions without judgment can help you manage them more effectively.

1. **Acknowledge Your Feelings:**
   - **Name Your Emotions:** Identifying what you are feeling can be the first step toward understanding and managing your emotions. For example, "I feel sad," or "I feel frustrated."
   - **Accept Without Judgment:** Allow yourself to feel your emotions without labeling them as good or bad. Acceptance can help reduce the intensity of negative emotions.
2. **Observe Without Reacting:**
   - **Mindful Observation:** Observe your emotions as they arise, without immediately reacting to them. This can give you the space to choose how to respond.
   - **Create a Pause:** When you notice a strong emotion, take a moment to breathe deeply before responding. This pause can prevent reactive behavior and promote thoughtful responses.

8.2 Practicing Self-Compassion

Self-compassion involves treating yourself with kindness and understanding during difficult times. It can help you cope with the challenges of living with PSP or caring for someone with PSP.

1. **Be Kind to Yourself:**
   - **Positive Self-Talk:** Replace self-criticism with supportive and encouraging words. For example, instead of saying, "I should be handling this better," try, "I am doing my best in a difficult situation."
   - **Practice Forgiveness:** Forgive yourself for mistakes or perceived shortcomings. Understand that everyone has limitations and it's okay to have moments of struggle.
2. **Self-Care Practices:**
   - **Physical Self-Care:** Ensure you are taking care of your physical needs, such as eating well, getting enough sleep, and exercising regularly.
   - **Emotional Self-Care:** Engage in activities that bring you joy and relaxation, such as reading, listening to music, or spending time in nature.
3. **Mindful Self-Compassion Exercises:**
   - **Self-Compassion Break:** When you are feeling stressed or upset, take a moment to acknowledge your suffering, remind yourself that suffering is a part of life, and

offer yourself words of kindness and
support.

- **Loving-Kindness Meditation:** Use phrases like, "May I be happy. May I be healthy. May I be safe. May I live with ease," to cultivate self-compassion.

8.3 Gratitude and Positive Thinking

Cultivating gratitude and positive thinking can significantly enhance emotional well-being. It helps shift focus from what is lacking or challenging to what is appreciated and positive.

1. **Daily Gratitude Practice:**
   - **Gratitude Journal:** Keep a journal where you write down three things you are grateful for each day. This practice can help shift your focus to the positive aspects of your life.
   - **Gratitude Rituals:** Incorporate gratitude into your daily routine, such as expressing gratitude before meals or before going to bed.
2. **Positive Affirmations:**
   - **Create Affirmations:** Develop a set of positive affirmations that resonate with you, such as, "I am strong," "I am capable," or "I am worthy of love."

- **Repeat Daily:** Repeat these affirmations daily, especially during challenging times, to reinforce positive thinking and self-belief.

3. **Reframe Negative Thoughts:**
   - **Identify Negative Thoughts:** Pay attention to negative thoughts and patterns. Challenge their validity and consider alternative, more positive perspectives.
   - **Replace with Positive Thoughts:** Consciously replace negative thoughts with positive ones. For example, change "I can't handle this" to "I am finding ways to cope and manage."

By recognizing and accepting emotions, practicing self-compassion, and cultivating gratitude and positive thinking, PSP patients and caregivers can enhance their emotional well-being and build resilience. The next chapter will focus on specific mindfulness practices designed for caregivers, providing further support for those in a caregiving role.

Chapter 9: Mindfulness for Caregivers

9.1 The Caregiver's Role

Caregivers play a crucial role in supporting PSP patients, often balancing multiple responsibilities and experiencing significant emotional and physical strain. Understanding the importance of self-care and mindfulness can help caregivers maintain their well-being while providing the best possible care.

- **Emotional Challenges:** Caregivers may experience feelings of guilt, frustration, sadness, and helplessness. Acknowledging these emotions and finding healthy ways to cope is essential.
- **Physical Demands:** The physical tasks of caregiving can be exhausting. Ensuring caregivers take care of their own health is vital to sustain their ability to care for others.
- **Balancing Responsibilities:** Juggling caregiving duties with personal and professional responsibilities can lead to burnout. Mindfulness can help caregivers manage stress and maintain balance.

9.2 Self-Care for Caregivers

Self-care is not a luxury but a necessity for caregivers. Taking time for self-care can prevent burnout and improve the quality of care provided to PSP patients.

1. **Daily Self-Care Practices:**
    *   **Set Aside Time for Yourself:** Schedule regular breaks and time for activities you enjoy, such as reading, walking, or hobbies.
    *   **Maintain Physical Health:** Prioritize regular exercise, a balanced diet, and sufficient sleep. These are fundamental to maintaining energy and resilience.
    *   **Emotional Support:** Seek support from friends, family, or support groups. Sharing your experiences and feelings can provide relief and perspective.
2. **Mindful Self-Care Techniques:**
    *   **Mindful Breathing:** Practice mindful breathing exercises to calm your mind and reduce stress. Even a few minutes of deep breathing can make a significant difference.
    *   **Body Scan Meditation:** Use body scan meditation to check in with your body, release tension, and promote relaxation.
    *   **Gratitude Practice:** Incorporate gratitude exercises into your daily routine to focus on positive aspects of your life.
3. **Professional Help:**
    *   **Counseling and Therapy:** Consider seeking professional counseling or therapy to address emotional challenges and develop coping strategies.
    *   **Respite Care:** Utilize respite care services to take breaks and recharge, knowing your loved one is in good hands.

9.3 Building a Support System

A strong support system is essential for caregivers. Connecting with others who understand your experiences can provide emotional support, practical advice, and a sense of community.

1. **Family and Friends:**
   - **Communicate Needs:** Clearly communicate your needs and ask for help when necessary. Friends and family are often willing to support but may not know how.
   - **Involve Loved Ones:** Encourage family members to take part in caregiving tasks, creating a shared responsibility and reducing your burden.
2. **Support Groups:**
   - **Join Support Groups:** Participate in local or online support groups for caregivers of PSP patients. Sharing experiences with others facing similar challenges can be comforting and informative.
   - **Peer Support:** Build relationships with other caregivers who can offer empathy, advice, and a listening ear.
3. **Professional Networks:**
   - **Healthcare Providers:** Maintain open communication with healthcare providers. They can offer guidance, resources, and support tailored to your loved one's needs.

- **Community Resources:** Utilize community resources such as caregiver programs, workshops, and respite services to enhance your support network.

By prioritizing self-care, practicing mindfulness, and building a robust support system, caregivers can enhance their well-being and provide better care for PSP patients. The next chapter will focus on integrating mindfulness into daily life, offering practical tips and techniques for seamless incorporation of mindfulness practices.

Chapter 10: Integrating Mindfulness into Daily Life

10.1 Mindful Eating

Mindful eating involves paying full attention to the experience of eating and drinking, both inside and outside the body. This practice can help improve digestion, foster a healthy relationship with food, and promote a sense of peace and satisfaction.

1. **Engage Your Senses:**
   - **Notice Colors and Textures:** Before you start eating, take a moment to observe the colors, shapes, and textures of your food.
   - **Smell the Aroma:** Inhale the aromas and notice any sensations that arise.
   - **Taste Mindfully:** Take small bites and chew slowly, savoring the flavors. Pay attention to the taste and texture of each bite.
2. **Eat Without Distractions:**
   - **Create a Calm Environment:** Turn off the TV, put away your phone, and minimize other distractions during meals.
   - **Focus on Eating:** Concentrate on the act of eating and the sensations it brings. This can help you feel more satisfied and prevent overeating.
3. **Listen to Your Body:**
   - **Recognize Hunger and Fullness:** Pay attention to your body's hunger and

fullness signals. Eat when you're hungry and stop when you're satisfied.

- **Avoid Emotional Eating:** Be mindful of emotional triggers that may lead to eating when not hungry. Use mindfulness techniques to address emotional needs.

10.2 Daily Mindfulness Activities

Incorporating mindfulness into everyday activities can help you stay present and reduce stress throughout the day. Here are some practical ways to integrate mindfulness into daily life:

1. **Mindful Walking:**
   - **Focus on Your Steps:** Pay attention to the sensation of your feet touching the ground and the movement of your body as you walk.
   - **Observe Your Surroundings:** Notice the sights, sounds, and smells around you. Engage with the environment without judgment.
2. **Mindful Housework:**
   - **Be Present:** Focus on the task at hand, whether it's washing dishes, sweeping, or folding laundry. Pay attention to the sensations and movements involved.
   - **Practice Gratitude:** Use housework as an opportunity to practice gratitude for your home and the ability to care for it.

3. **Mindful Communication:**
    - **Listen Fully:** When talking to someone, give them your full attention. Listen without interrupting and respond thoughtfully.
    - **Express Mindfully:** Choose your words carefully and express yourself with clarity and kindness.
4. **Mindful Relaxation:**
    - **Take Short Breaks:** Throughout the day, take short breaks to practice mindful breathing or stretching. These moments of relaxation can help reduce stress and improve focus.
    - **Engage in Relaxing Activities:** Spend time on activities that promote relaxation, such as reading, listening to music, or spending time in nature.

10.3 Sustaining Your Practice

Maintaining a consistent mindfulness practice can be challenging, but with persistence and dedication, it can become a natural part of your daily routine. Here are some tips for sustaining your mindfulness practice:

1. **Set Realistic Goals:**
    - **Start Small:** Begin with short, manageable sessions of mindfulness practice and gradually increase the duration as you become more comfortable.

- **Be Patient:** Understand that building a mindfulness practice takes time and patience. Be kind to yourself and celebrate your progress.

2. **Create a Routine:**
   - **Schedule Practice Time:** Set aside specific times each day for mindfulness practice. Consistency can help reinforce the habit.
   - **Incorporate into Daily Activities:** Integrate mindfulness into your daily activities, such as eating, walking, and communicating.

3. **Stay Motivated:**
   - **Reflect on Benefits:** Regularly reflect on the benefits you experience from your mindfulness practice, such as reduced stress and improved well-being.
   - **Join a Community:** Consider joining a mindfulness group or community for support, motivation, and accountability.

4. **Adapt and Adjust:**
   - **Be Flexible:** Allow your practice to evolve and adapt to your changing needs and circumstances. If a particular technique no longer serves you, try a new one.
   - **Practice Self-Compassion:** Be gentle with yourself if you miss a practice session. Instead of feeling discouraged, recommit to your practice with renewed intention.

By integrating mindfulness into daily activities and sustaining a consistent practice, PSP patients and caregivers can enhance their overall quality of life and build resilience. The next chapter will provide resources and further reading to support your mindfulness journey.

Chapter 11: Resources and Further Reading

11.1 Recommended Books and Articles

Exploring additional resources can deepen your understanding of mindfulness and provide further techniques and insights tailored to your needs. Here are some highly recommended books and articles:

1. **Books:**
   - **"The Miracle of Mindfulness" by Thich Nhat Hanh:**
     - A classic guide to mindfulness, offering practical exercises and insights into the practice of being present.
   - **"Wherever You Go, There You Are" by Jon Kabat-Zinn:**
     - An accessible introduction to mindfulness meditation by one of the pioneers in the field.
   - **"Full Catastrophe Living" by Jon Kabat-Zinn:**
     - A comprehensive guide to using mindfulness to manage stress, pain, and illness.
   - **"Radical Acceptance" by Tara Brach:**
     - Explores how to embrace yourself and your life with the heart of a Buddha.

- **"The Mindful Path to Self-Compassion" by Christopher Germer:**
  - Provides a step-by-step program for transforming your relationship with yourself.

2. **Articles:**
   - **"What Is Mindfulness?" by Greater Good Science Center:**
     - An overview of mindfulness and its benefits, with links to related research.
   - **"How Mindfulness Can Help Caregivers" by Mayo Clinic:**
     - Discusses the benefits of mindfulness for caregivers and offers practical tips.
   - **"Mindfulness for Anxiety and Depression" by Harvard Health:**
     - Examines how mindfulness practices can help manage anxiety and depression.

11.2 Online Resources and Apps

Leveraging technology can make mindfulness practices more accessible and convenient. Here are some online resources and apps to support your mindfulness journey:

1. **Websites:**
   - **Mindful.org:**
     - Offers a wealth of articles, guided meditations, and resources on mindfulness and meditation.
   - **Insight Timer:**
     - Provides free guided meditations, courses, and a community of meditators.
   - **Headspace:**
     - Features guided meditations, courses, and tips for integrating mindfulness into daily life (subscription-based).
2. **Apps:**
   - **Calm:**
     - Offers guided meditations, sleep stories, and relaxation techniques (subscription-based).
   - **10% Happier:**
     - Provides practical meditation techniques and teachings (subscription-based).
   - **Breathe2Relax:**
     - A free app focusing on breathing exercises to manage stress.

11.3 Support Groups and Communities

Connecting with others who share similar experiences can provide valuable support and encouragement. Here are some options for finding support groups and communities:

1. **In-Person Support Groups:**
   - **Local Community Centers:**
     - Check with local community centers, hospitals, or health organizations for mindfulness or caregiver support groups.
   - **Hospice and Palliative Care Organizations:**
     - Many hospice and palliative care organizations offer support groups for caregivers.
2. **Online Support Groups:**
   - **Facebook Groups:**
     - Search for Facebook groups focused on mindfulness, PSP, or caregiver support. These groups can provide a platform to share experiences, ask questions, and receive support.
   - **Reddit Communities:**
     - Subreddits like r/mindfulness, r/caregivers, and r/ProgressiveSupranuclearPalsy offer communities for sharing and support.
3. **Professional Organizations:**
   - **The Mindfulness Association:**
     - Offers courses, resources, and a community for mindfulness practitioners.
   - **The Caregiver Action Network:**

- Provides resources and support for caregivers, including online forums and articles.

By exploring these resources, PSP patients and caregivers can continue to deepen their mindfulness practice, access valuable support, and stay informed about new techniques and research. The final chapter will include personal stories and testimonials, offering inspiration and insights from those who have integrated mindfulness into their lives.

Chapter 12: Personal Stories and Testimonials

12.1 Experiences of PSP Patients

Hearing from others who are living with Progressive Supranuclear Palsy (PSP) can provide invaluable insights and inspiration. These stories highlight the resilience, courage, and mindfulness practices that have helped them navigate their journeys.

John's Story:

- **Background:** Diagnosed with PSP five years ago, John initially struggled with the physical and emotional toll of the disease.
- **Mindfulness Practice:** John started practicing mindfulness meditation after a friend recommended it. He found that focusing on his breath and using body scan techniques helped him manage his anxiety and reduce muscle tension.
- **Impact:** Mindfulness has allowed John to stay present and appreciate the small joys in life. He now leads a local support group, sharing his experiences and teaching mindfulness techniques to others with PSP.

Mary's Story:

- **Background:** Mary, a retired teacher, was diagnosed with PSP three years ago. The progressive symptoms caused significant frustration and fear.

- **Mindfulness Practice:** Mary incorporated mindful walking and gratitude journaling into her daily routine. She found that these practices helped her stay connected to the present moment and find peace amidst her challenges.
- **Impact:** Mary reports feeling more grounded and less overwhelmed. Her mindfulness practice has strengthened her relationships with family and friends, as she communicates more openly and mindfully.

12.2 Caregiver Insights

Caregivers play a critical role in supporting PSP patients, often facing their own set of challenges. These stories from caregivers demonstrate the power of mindfulness in enhancing their well-being and caregiving abilities.

Linda's Story:

- **Background:** Linda has been caring for her husband, who was diagnosed with PSP four years ago. The demands of caregiving left her feeling exhausted and emotionally drained.
- **Mindfulness Practice:** Linda began practicing mindful breathing and meditation. She also joined an online mindfulness community for caregivers, where she found support and encouragement.
- **Impact:** Mindfulness has helped Linda manage her stress and prevent burnout. She feels more

patient and compassionate, both towards herself and her husband. Linda now encourages other caregivers to explore mindfulness as a tool for self-care.

Mark's Story:

- **Background:** Mark, a father of two, became the primary caregiver for his mother after her PSP diagnosis. Balancing caregiving with his professional and personal responsibilities was overwhelming.
- **Mindfulness Practice:** Mark started using guided meditations and mindfulness apps to find moments of calm throughout his day. He also practiced mindful communication with his mother, improving their interactions.
- **Impact:** Mindfulness has given Mark a sense of control and peace. He feels more connected to his mother and better equipped to handle the challenges of caregiving. Mark shares his mindfulness journey with other caregivers, advocating for its benefits.

12.3 Lessons Learned and Inspirational Stories

These inspirational stories illustrate the profound impact mindfulness can have on the lives of PSP patients and their caregivers. The lessons learned from their experiences can offer guidance and motivation to others on similar paths.

Alice's Journey:

- **Background:** Alice, diagnosed with PSP six years ago, found herself battling depression and isolation.
- **Lesson Learned:** Mindfulness taught Alice to accept her emotions without judgment. She learned to embrace her feelings of sadness and fear, which ultimately reduced their power over her.
- **Inspiration:** Alice's story highlights the importance of self-compassion and acceptance. By embracing mindfulness, she has found a renewed sense of purpose and joy in her life.

Tom and Sarah's Journey:

- **Background:** Tom, diagnosed with PSP, and his wife Sarah faced the challenges of the disease together. They struggled with communication and emotional strain.
- **Lesson Learned:** Through mindful communication and joint mindfulness practices, Tom and Sarah improved their relationship and mutual understanding. They learned to support each other more effectively.
- **Inspiration:** Their journey underscores the power of mindfulness in strengthening relationships and fostering empathy. Tom and Sarah's story inspires other couples to explore mindfulness as a way to navigate the challenges of PSP together.

These personal stories and testimonials demonstrate the transformative potential of mindfulness for PSP patients and their caregivers. By sharing their experiences, they offer hope, encouragement, and practical insights for integrating mindfulness into daily life.

This concludes our exploration of mindfulness practices tailored to the needs of PSP patients and their caregivers. We hope this book serves as a valuable resource, providing tools, techniques, and inspiration to enhance your well-being and navigate the challenges of PSP with resilience and grace.

Conclusion

Embracing Mindfulness in the Journey with PSP

Living with Progressive Supranuclear Palsy (PSP) presents numerous challenges for both patients and caregivers. The journey can be fraught with emotional, physical, and psychological hurdles. However, integrating mindfulness practices into daily life offers a powerful way to manage these challenges, enhancing overall well-being and fostering a sense of peace and resilience.

Key Takeaways

1. **Understanding Mindfulness:**
   - Mindfulness is about being fully present in the moment, observing thoughts and emotions without judgment, and fostering a sense of calm and clarity.
2. **Practical Techniques:**
   - Incorporate mindful breathing, meditation, body awareness, and mindful movement into your routine to manage stress and improve emotional well-being.
3. **Daily Integration:**
   - Integrate mindfulness into everyday activities, such as eating, walking, and communication, to maintain a consistent practice and stay grounded.

4. **Self-Care for Caregivers:**
    - Prioritize self-care and build a robust support system to prevent burnout and enhance caregiving abilities.
5. **Resources and Support:**
    - Utilize books, articles, online resources, apps, and support groups to deepen your mindfulness practice and find community support.

The Transformative Power of Mindfulness

By embracing mindfulness, PSP patients and caregivers can transform their experience of the disease. Mindfulness offers a path to:

- **Reduced Stress and Anxiety:** Through regular practice, you can lower stress levels and manage anxiety more effectively.
- **Enhanced Emotional Well-Being:** Mindfulness fosters emotional resilience, helping you navigate the emotional challenges of PSP with greater ease.
- **Improved Physical Health:** Techniques such as mindful movement and body scan meditation can alleviate physical tension and promote relaxation.
- **Stronger Relationships:** Mindful communication can improve understanding and connection between patients and caregivers, strengthening relationships.

Moving Forward with Hope and Resilience

As you continue your journey with PSP, remember that mindfulness is a practice that evolves over time. Be patient with yourself and celebrate small victories along the way. The stories and techniques shared in this book are meant to inspire and guide you, providing practical tools to enhance your quality of life.

Final Words

We hope this book has provided valuable insights and practical guidance for incorporating mindfulness into your life. Remember, you are not alone on this journey. By embracing mindfulness, you can cultivate a sense of peace, resilience, and hope, navigating the challenges of PSP with grace and strength.

Thank you for embarking on this mindfulness journey with us. May you find comfort, support, and inspiration in the practices and stories shared in this book.

Resources and References:

For further reading and exploration, please refer to the resources and references provided in Chapter 11. These materials offer additional guidance and support for your mindfulness practice.

This concludes the book "Mindfulness and PSP: Techniques for Coping." We wish you peace, strength, and mindfulness on your journey.

About the Author: Laura Louizos

Laura Louizos is a compassionate advocate and caregiver who founded the Coleen Cunningham Foundation in honor of her mother, Coleen Cunningham, who bravely battled Progressive Supranuclear Palsy (PSP). Throughout her mother's journey, Laura was her primary caregiver, experiencing firsthand the challenges and triumphs that come with caring for a loved one with a neurodegenerative disease.

Inspired by her mother's strength and resilience, Laura dedicated herself to supporting families and individuals affected by PSP. The Coleen Cunningham Foundation focuses on providing comprehensive support, respite care, and resources to help families navigate the complexities of living with PSP. Laura's work is centered on ensuring that no family faces this journey alone, offering emotional and practical support at every step.

No One Walks Alone

For resources and support visit:

pspawareness.com